MACROBIOTIC COOKBOOK

MAIN COURSE - 60+ Breakfast, Lunch, Dinner and Dessert Recipes for high energy and clear thinking

TABLE OF CONTENTS

BREAKFAST 7

SCRAMBLED TOFU 7

PORRDIGE 9

MISO APPLE CRUMBLE 10

BUCKWHEAT BRETON GALETTES 12

BUCKWHEAT PANCAKES 14

MACROBIOTIC BREAKFAST 16

BROWN RICE PANCAKES 17

BEAN HUMMUS 18

MILLET PUDDING 19

PUMPKIN OATMEAL 20

CHIA PUDDING WITH NUTS 22

MOCHI CROUTONS 24

NISHIME VEGETABLES 25

RICE PORRIDGE 26

BROWN RICE BOWL 28

QUINOA FALAFEL 29

MORNING LOADED SWEET POTATO 31

TOFU BACON 33

SIMPLE PANCAKES 35

BANANA& RASPBERRIES PANCAKES 36

LUNCH 39

QUINOA FALAFEL 39

VEGAN RAMEN 41

ROASTED CAULIFLOWER 43

GARLIC TOFU 45

BUDDHA BOWL 47

VEGAN RICE BACON 49

FALAFEL BITES 51

ZUCCHINI FRIES 53

ZUCCHINI DAL 55

CHICKPEA PATTIES 57

GAZPACHO SALAD 59

RADISH & PARSLEY SALAD 60

ZUCCHINI & BELL PEPPER SALAD 61

QUINOA & AVOCADO SALAD 62

TOFU SALAD 64

PAD THAI SALAD 65

AVOCADO SALAD 66

MUSHROOM SALAD 67

MIXED GREENS SALAD 68

QUINOA SALAD 69

DINNER 71

ONION SOUP 71

ZUCCHINI SOUP 73

SAUERKRAUT SOUP 75

GREEK RICE SOUP 77

GAZPACHO 79

TORTELLINI SOUP 81

LEBANESE SOUP 83

BROCCOLI SOUP 85

SWEET POTATO SOUP 87

VEGAN PHO 89

SMOOTHIES 91

MACROBIOTIC SMOOTHIE.. 91

PALEO SMOOTHIE 92

MORNING CHOCHOLATE SMOOTHIE 93

ALKALINE SMOOTHIE 94

SIMPLE MACROBIOTIC SMOOTHIE 95

ENERGY BOOSTING SMOOTHIE 96

TURMERIC SMOOTHIE.. 97

PINEAPPLE SMOOTHIE 98

KIWI-KALE SMOOTHIE 99

STRAWBERRY SMOOTHIE 100

Copyright 2019 by Noah Jerris - All rights reserved.

This document is geared towards providing exact and reliable information in regards to the topic and issue covered. The publication is sold with the idea that the publisher is not required to render accounting, officially permitted, or otherwise, qualified services. If advice is necessary, legal or professional, a practiced individual in the profession should be ordered.

- From a Declaration of Principles which was accepted and approved equally by a Committee of the American Bar Association and a Committee of Publishers and Associations.

In no way is it legal to reproduce, duplicate, or transmit any part of this document in either electronic means or in printed format. Recording of this publication is strictly prohibited and any storage of this document is not allowed unless with written permission from the publisher. All rights reserved.

The information provided herein is stated to be truthful and consistent, in that any liability, in terms of inattention or otherwise, by any usage or abuse of any policies, processes, or directions contained within is the solitary and utter responsibility of the recipient reader. Under no circumstances will any legal responsibility or blame be held against the publisher for any reparation, damages, or monetary loss due to the information herein, either directly or indirectly.

Respective authors own all copyrights not held by the publisher.

The information herein is offered for informational

purposes solely, and is universal as so. The presentation of the information is without contract or any type of guarantee assurance.

The trademarks that are used are without any consent, and the publication of the trademark is without permission or backing by the trademark owner. All trademarks and brands within this book are for clarifying purposes only and are the owned by the owners themselves, not affiliated with this document.

Introduction

Macrobiotic recipes for personal enjoyment but also for family enjoyment. You will love them for sure for how easy it is to prepare them.

BREAKFAST

SCRAMBLED TOFU

Serves: **4**

Prep Time: **10** Minutes

Cook Time: **20** Minutes

Total Time: **30** Minutes

INGREDIENTS

- 2 lb. silken tofu
- 1 tablespoon olive oil
- 2 tsp curry powder
- 2 tsp turmeric powder
- ½ lime juice
- ¼ lb. kale leaves
- 1 onion

DIRECTIONS

1. In a pan heat olive oil, add onion, kale leaves, salt and cook for 2-3 minutes

2. Add remaining ingredients and cook until tofu is soft
3. When ready remove from heat and serve with lime juice

PORRDIGE

Serves: 2
Prep Time: 5 Minutes
Cook Time: 15 Minutes
Total Time: 20 Minutes

INGREDIENTS

- ¼ cup oats
- 1 cup water
- pinch of salt

TOPPINGS

- 1 tablespoon black sugar
- 1 tablespoon coconut flakes
- 1 tablespoon berries

DIRECTIONS

1. In a pot add oats, water, salt and bring to a boil
2. Simmer on low heat for 12-15 minutes
3. When ready pour the porridge into a bowl
4. Top with coconut flakes or berries and serve

MISO APPLE CRUMBLE

Serves: **4**

Prep Time: **10** Minutes

Cook Time: **20** Minutes

Total Time: **30** Minutes

INGREDIENTS

- 2 tablespoons white miso
- 2 oz. brown sugar
- 200 ml coconut milk
- 2 apples
- 3 oz. porridge
- 2 oz. cranberries

DIRECTIONS

1. In a saucepan add coconut milk and sugar
2. Stir well add miso and cook until sugar has melted
3. Add apple slices and to the caramel sauce and simmer on low heat

4. In a pan cook the oats and seeds and portion into 2 bowls
5. Pour the sauce over and mix well
6. Serve when ready

BUCKWHEAT BRETON GALETTES

Serves: **4**

Prep Time: **10** Minutes

Cook Time: **15** Minutes

Total Time: **25** Minutes

INGREDIENTS

- 1 tablespoon flax seeds
- ¼ lb. buckwheat flour
- 150 ml plant milk
- 300 ml water

TOPPING

- 1 tablespoon sesame oil
- 1 apple
- 4 apricots
- 1 tablespoon maple syrup

DIRECTIONS

1. Place the chia seeds into a bowl, add water and mix well

2. In another bowl add buckwheat flour, milk, chia seeds mixture and mix
3. In a frying pan pour ¼ of the mixture and cook for 2-3 minutes per side
4. When ready remove pancakes to a plate
5. Fry apricots and apple slices until soft
6. Serve with the pancakes and maple syrup

BUCKWHEAT PANCAKES

Serves: **6**

Prep Time: **5** Minutes

Cook Time: **15** Minutes

Total Time: **20** Minutes

INGREDIENTS

- 3 oz. buckwheat flour
- ¼ lb. apple puree
- 2 oz. walnuts
- 1 banana
- 1 tablespoon olive oil
- maple syrup

DIRECTIONS

1. In a blender add all ingredients for the pancakes and blend until smooth
2. In a frying pan heat olive oil and pour 1/6 of the batter
3. Cook for 1-2 minutes per side

4. When ready remove from the pan and serve with apple puree

MACROBIOTIC BREAKFAST

Serves: 2
Prep Time: 5 Minutes
Cook Time: 15 Minutes
Total Time: 20 Minutes

INGREDIENTS

- ¼ cup brown rice
- ½ cup kale
- ¼ cup spinach
- 1 tsp tamari
- 1 tsp plum vinegar
- ¼ avocado

DIRECTIONS

1. In a pot add water, broccoli and cook covered for 2-3 minutes
2. Add greens, rice, vinegar, brown rice and tamari
3. Cook for another 4-5 minutes
4. When ready transfer to a bowl, top with avocado slices and serve

BROWN RICE PANCAKES

Serves: *8*

Prep Time: *5* Minutes

Cook Time: *15* Minutes

Total Time: *20* Minutes

INGREDIENTS

- 250 ml coconut milk
- 1 tsp baking powder
- 300g brown rice flour
- 2 tablespoons olive oil
- blueberries

DIRECTIONS

1. In a blender add all the ingredients except blueberries and blend until smooth
2. In a frying pan heat olive oil and pour 1/8 batter and cook for 1-2 minutes per side
3. When ready remove from the pan and serve with blueberries on top

BEAN HUMMUS

Serves: **4**

Prep Time: **5** Minutes

Cook Time: **15** Minutes

Total Time: **20** Minutes

INGREDIENTS

- 2 cans white beans
- 2 tablespoons tahini paste
- 2 garlic cloves
- 2 tablespoons olive oil
- 2 tablespoons flax seeds

DIRECTIONS

1. In a blender add all ingredients together and blend until smooth
2. Add water if needed and blend until beans are smooth
3. Toast the seeds and sprinkle over the bean hummus, drizzle olive oil and serve

MILLET PUDDING

Serves: **4**

Prep Time: **10** Minutes

Cook Time: **25** Minutes

Total Time: **35** Minutes

INGREDIENTS

- 3 cups non-diary milk
- ¼ cup millet
- 1 tsp vanilla extract
- ¼ tsp almond extract
- ¼ tsp cinnamon
- almonds

DIRECTIONS

1. In a pot add the millet and toast well
2. Add remaining ingredients to the pot and stir to combine
3. Bring to a boil and simmer for 18-20 minutes
4. When ready remove from heat and sprinkle almonds or blueberries

PUMPKIN OATMEAL

Serves: **4**

Prep Time: **5** Minutes

Cook Time: **15** Minutes

Total Time: **20** Minutes

INGREDIENTS

- ¼ cup oats
- ¼ cup almond milk
- ¼ cup water
- 1 tablespoon butter
- ½ cup pumpkin puree
- 1 tablespoon maple syrup
- 1 banana
- 1 tablespoon walnuts

DIRECTIONS

1. **In a saucepan combine water, oats, milk, salt and bring to a boil**

2. Simmer for 8-10 minutes and stir in pumpkin puree, butter and cook until the butter is fully melted
3. When ready top with remaining ingredients and serve

CHIA PUDDING WITH NUTS

Serves: **1**

Prep Time: **10** Minutes

Cook Time: **10** Minutes

Total Time: **20** Minutes

INGREDIENTS

- 3 tablespoons wheat flakes
- 2 tablespoons nuts
- 1 tablespoon carob powder
- 1 tsp honey
- 1 banana
- 1 tablespoon chia seeds

DIRECTIONS

1. In a bowl place wheat flakes and soak in water overnight
2. In a blender add chia seeds, honey, carob powder, banana and blend until smooth
3. Combine the mixture with soaked wheat flakes and mix well

4. Add dry fruits, mix well and serve

MOCHI CROUTONS

Serves: **4**

Prep Time: **5** Minutes

Cook Time: **5** Minutes

Total Time: **10** Minutes

INGREDIENTS

- ¼ package mocha
- 1 tablespoon sesame oil

DIRECTIONS

1. In an iron skillet add mochi cubes
2. Add sesame oil and cook on low heat for 2-3 minutes
3. When ready remove from heat and serve with miso soup

NISHIME VEGETABLES

Serves: **4**
Prep Time: **10** Minutes
Cook Time: **20** Minutes
Total Time: **30** Minutes

INGREDIENTS

- 1 cup squash
- 1 cup carrots
- 1 cup green cabbage
- 1-inch kombu
- ¼ cup tamari
- ¼ cup water

DIRECTIONS

1. In a pot add vegetables and sprinkle salt
2. Add water and bring to a boil, simmer for 15-20 minutes
3. When ready sprinkle salt and remove from the heat
4. Serve when ready

RICE PORRIDGE

Serves: 2
Prep Time: **10** Minutes
Cook Time: **50** Minutes
Total Time: **60** Minutes

INGREDIENTS

- 1 cup brown rice
- 2 cups water
- pinch of salt
- 1 cup apricots
- 1 handful sunflower seeds

DIRECTIONS

1. In a bowl cover rice with water and let it soak overnight
2. Place the rice in a pan, add water and bring to a boil
3. Add salt and simmer on low heat for 45-50 minutes
4. Stir well and place the rice into bowls

5. Serve with sunflower seeds and apricots

BROWN RICE BOWL

Serves: **4**
Prep Time: **5** Minutes
Cook Time: **15** Minutes
Total Time: **20** Minutes

INGREDIENTS

- ¼ cup cooked brown rice
- 1 cup greens
- 1 tsp tamari
- 1 tsp plum vinegar
- ¼ avocado

DIRECTIONS

1. In a pot add broccoli, water and bring to a boil
2. Add greens, tamari, vinegar, brown rice and cook for another 4-5 minutes
3. When ready transfer to a bowl, top with avocado slices and serve

QUINOA FALAFEL

Serves: **8-12**

Prep Time: **15** Minutes

Cook Time: **15** Minutes

Total Time: **30** Minutes

INGREDIENTS

- 2 cups quinoa
- 2 cups chickpea
- 1 onion
- 1 tablespoon tahini
- 4 garlic cloves
- 1 cup parsley
- 2 tsp salt
- 2 tsp cumin
- 1 tsp coriander
- 2 tablespoons olive oil
- 1 tablespoon cornstarch
- 1 tablespoon lemon juice
- 1 cup water

DIRECTIONS

1. In a blender add parsley, coriander, garlic, lemon juice, onion, water and blend until smooth
2. Add the rest of the ingredients and blend again
3. Transfer mixture to a bowl, form small patties from the mixture
4. Place the patties in the freezer for a couple of minutes
5. In a pan heat olive oil and fry the patties for 2-3 minutes per side
6. When ready remove patties from the pan and serve

MORNING LOADED SWEET POTATO

Serves: 2

Prep Time: 15 Minutes

Cook Time: 15 Minutes

Total Time: 30 Minutes

INGREDIENTS

- 2 sweet potatoes
- 2 tablespoons veggie stock
- ¼ cup cooked rice
- ¼ cup smoked tofu
- 1 onion
- 1 garlic clove
- 1 tsp red pepper flakes
- ¼ tsp cumin
- ¼ tsp oregano

TOPPING

- 1 tablespoon cheddar cheese

DIRECTIONS

1. In a microwave bake the potatoes until soft
2. In a skillet sauté onion, red pepper flakes, tofu, oregano, cumin and stir well
3. Add veggie stock, salt and cook for another 4-5 minutes
4. Cut the potatoes lengthwise, mash them and add rice, tofu mixture and sprinkle cheddar cheese on top
5. Bake at 275 F for 8-10 minutes, when ready remove and serve

TOFU BACON

Serves: **6-8**

Prep Time: **15** Minutes

Cook Time: **10** Minutes

Total Time: **25** Minutes

INGREDIENTS

- 1 block tofu
- 1 tablespoon olive oil

MARINADE

- ¼ cup water
- 1 tablespoon coconut aminos
- 1 tablespoon brown sugar
- 1 tablespoon yeast
- 1 tsp tomato paste

DIRECTIONS

1. **Cut tofu into thin slices**
2. **In a bowl place all ingredients for the marinate and mix well**

3. Add tofu to the marinate and let it chill for a couple of minutes
4. In a skillet heat olive and fry tofu slices until crispy
5. When ready remove from the skillet and serve

SIMPLE PANCAKES

Serves: **4**

Prep Time: **5** Minutes

Cook Time: **15** Minutes

Total Time: **20** Minutes

INGREDIENTS

- 1 cup flour
- 2 tsp baking powder
- 1 tsp salt
- 1 tablespoon brown sugar
- 1 cup milk
- 1 egg
- 2 tablespoons butter

DIRECTIONS

1. In a bowl combine all ingredients together and mix well
2. In a skillet pour ¼ cup of the batter and fry each pancake for 1-2 minutes per side
3. When ready remove from the skillet and serve

BANANA& RASPBERRIES PANCAKES

Serves: **4**

Prep Time: **10** Minutes

Cook Time: **30** Minutes

Total Time: **40** Minutes

INGREDIENTS

- 1 cup soy milk
- 1 banana
- ½ cup raspberries
- 1 egg
- 1 tablespoons olive oil
- 1 cup almond flour
- 1 tsp baking power
- Maple syrup

DIRECTIONS

1. In a bowl combine all ingredients together, except raspberries, and mix well
2. In a skillet pour ¼ cup of the batter and fry each pancake for 1-2 minutes per side

3. When ready remove from the skillet and serve with maple syrup and raspberries on top

LUNCH

QUINOA FALAFEL

Serves: **6-8**

Prep Time: **15** Minutes

Cook Time: **25** Minutes

Total Time: **40** Minutes

INGREDIENTS

- 2 cups cooked quinoa
- 2 cups chickpeas
- 1 onion
- 1 tablespoon tahini
- 4 garlic cloves
- 1 cup parsley
- 2 tsp cumin
- 1 tsp coriander
- 2 tablespoons olive oil
- 1 tablespoon lemon juice

TAHINI SAUCE

- 1 cup water
- 1 cup tahini
- 1 garlic clove
- pinch of salt

DIRECTIONS

1. In a blender add garlic, parsley, coriander, lemon juice, onion and blend until smooth
2. Add the remaining ingredients and blend again
3. Form patties and freeze patties for 15-20 minutes
4. In a frying pan place the patties and fry until golden brown
5. When ready transfer patties to a plate and serve with tahini sauce

VEGAN RAMEN

Serves: **6**

Prep Time: **10** Minutes

Cook Time: **20** Minutes

Total Time: **30** Minutes

INGREDIENTS

- 4 cups vegetable broth
- 2 tablespoon soy sauce
- 2 clove garlic
- 1 tsp miso paste
- 1 cup mushrooms
- 1 cup tofu
- 1 cup broccoli florets
- 1 cup ramen noodles
- 1 cup sprouts
- ½ red onion
- ¼ cup cilantro
- 1 tablespoon sesame seeds

DIRECTIONS

1. In a pan sauté garlic, onion and set aside
2. In a pot add broth and sautéed onion, garlic and stir in miso paste
3. Transfer everything to a blender and blend until smooth
4. Add salt soy sauce and blend again
5. In a pan fry mushrooms, noodles, broccoli, sprouts, and tofu
6. Stir in broth and sesame seeds
7. When ready serve fried vegetables with the garlic mixture

ROASTED CAULIFLOWER

Serves: 2

Prep Time: **10** Minutes

Cook Time: **30** Minutes

Total Time: **40** Minutes

INGREDIENTS

- 1 cauliflower head

BBQ SAUCE

- ¼ cup tomato sauce
- 1 tsp garam masala
- 1 tablespoon peanut butter
- 1 tsp olive oil
- 1 tsp Worchester sauce
- 1 tsp soy sauce
- 1 clove garlic
- 1 black pepper

DIRECTIONS

1. In a bowl combine all ingredients for the sauce and whisk well
2. Place the cauliflower in a baking dish and bake for 20-25 minutes at 225 F or until brown
3. When ready remove from the oven and serve with bbq sauce

GARLIC TOFU

Serves: **4**

Prep Time: **10** Minutes

Cook Time: **20** Minutes

Total Time: **30** Minutes

INGREDIENTS

- 1 cup tofu
- 1 cup cooked brown rice
- 1 tablespoon chives
- 1 tablespoon olive oil
- 1 tsp vegan butter
- ¼ cup hoisin sauce
- 1 tablespoon soy sauce
- 2 cloves garlic
- 1 tsp sesame seeds

DIRECTIONS

1. In a bowl combine hoisin sauce, garlic and mix well

2. Add tofu, toss well and refrigerate overnight
3. In a skillet heat olive oil and add tofu and spread on a single layer
4. Add remaining ingredients, sprinkle sesame seeds and cook until browned
5. When ready remove from the pan and serve with brown rice

BUDDHA BOWL

Serves: **4**
Prep Time: **10** Minutes
Cook Time: **30** Minutes
Total Time: **40** Minutes

INGREDIENTS

- 1 cup buckwheat

DRESSING

- 1 tablespoon nutritional yeast
- 1 tsp mustard
- salt
- 1 clove garlic

DIRECTIONS

1. Place the buckwheat into a bowl and add 1-2 cups of water
2. In a blender all the ingredients for the dressing and blend until smooth

3. Divide the buckwheat between 2-3 plates and serve with dressing
4. Add toppings like tomatoes, bell pepper or radish sprouts

VEGAN RICE BACON

Serves: **4**

Prep Time: **10** Minutes

Cook Time: **30** Minutes

Total Time: **40** Minutes

INGREDIENTS

- 2 rice paper sheets
- 1 tablespoon water
- 1 tablespoon olive oil
- 1 tablespoon soy sauce
- ¼ tsp onion powder
- ¼ tsp cumin powder
- 1 tsp tomato sauce
- 1 tsp agave syrup

DIRECTIONS

1. In a bowl combine all ingredients together excepting the rice paper
2. Dip the rice paper into a large plate with water

3. Cut the paper into strips and lay the strips onto a baking tray
4. Brush with sauce from the blender and bake for 10-12 minutes at 300 F
5. When ready remove from the oven and serve

FALAFEL BITES

Serves: *12*

Prep Time: *5* Minutes

Cook Time: *15* Minutes

Total Time: *20* Minutes

INGREDIENTS

- 1 cup chickpeas
- 1 onion
- ¼ cup parsley
- 2 cloves garlic
- 1 tsp baking soda
- 1 tablespoon flour
- 1 tsp cumin
- ¼ tsp coriander

DIRECTIONS

1. In a blender add all the ingredients and blend until smooth
2. In a pan heat olive oil and form small patties

3. Cook each falafel until crispy
4. When ready remove and serve

ZUCCHINI FRIES

Serves: **6**

Prep Time: **10** Minutes

Cook Time: **20** Minutes

Total Time: **30** Minutes

INGREDIENTS

- 2 zucchinis
- ¼ cup breadcrumbs
- ¼ cup vegan cheese
- olive oil
- tahini
- pesto
- ketchup

DIRECTIONS

1. Cut zucchinis into thin strips
2. In a bowl add vegan cheese, breadcrumbs, salt and mix well
3. Dip each zucchini strip into the mixture

4. Place the strips onto a parchment paper
5. Bake for 18-20 minutes at 350 F
6. When ready remove from the oven and serve

ZUCCHINI DAL

Serves: 2
Prep Time: 5 Minutes
Cook Time: 20 Minutes
Total Time: 25 Minutes

INGREDIENTS

- 2 cups water
- ½ cup red lentils
- 1 zucchini
- 1 onion
- 2 tablespoons curry powder
- 1 tablespoon olive oil
- salt

DIRECTIONS

1. In a pot add zucchini, onion, pepper and sauté for 5-6 minutes
2. Ad lentils, water and the remaining ingredients
3. Cook on low heat for 15-18 minutes

4. When ready from heat, add scallions and serve

CHICKPEA PATTIES

Serves: **12**

Prep Time: **5** Minutes

Cook Time: **15** Minutes

Total Time: **20** Minutes

INGREDIENTS

- 2 lb. chickpeas
- ¼ cup parsley
- ½ red onion
- 2 tablespoons yeast flakes
- 2 tablespoons rosemary leaves
- olive oil

DIRECTIONS

1. Place chickpea in a blender and blend until smooth
2. Add remaining ingredients and blend again
3. Remove the mixture from the blender and form small patties

4. Heat olive oil in a pan and fry the patties for 2-3 minutes per side
5. When ready remove from the pan and serve

GAZPACHO SALAD

Serves: **4**
Prep Time: **10** Minutes

Cook Time: **30** Minutes

Total Time: **40** Minutes

INGREDIENTS

- ½ lb. cherry tomatoes
- ½ cucumber
- 3 oz. cooked quinoa
- 1 tsp bouillon powder
- 2 spring onions
- 1 red pepper
- ½ avocado
- 1 pack Japanese tofu

DIRECTIONS

1. **In a bowl combine all ingredients together**
2. **Add salad dressing, toss well and serve**

RADISH & PARSLEY SALAD

Serves: **4**

Prep Time: **10** Minutes

Cook Time: **30** Minutes

Total Time: **40** Minutes

INGREDIENTS

- 1 tsp olive oil
- ¼ lb. tomatoes
- 2 oz. radish
- 1 oz. parsley
- 1 tablespoon coriander
- salt

DIRECTIONS

1. In a bowl combine all ingredients together
2. Add salad dressing, toss well and serve

ZUCCHINI & BELL PEPPER SALAD

Serves: *1*
Prep Time: *5* Minutes
Cook Time: *5* Minutes
Total Time: *10* Minutes

INGREDIENTS

- ¼ cup zucchini
- ¼ cup red capsicum
- ½ cup yellow capsicum
- 1 cup sprouted moong
- ¼ cup apple
- 1 tablespoon olive oil
- 1 tsp lemon juice

DIRECTIONS

1. In a bowl combine all ingredients together
2. Add olive oil, toss well and serve

QUINOA & AVOCADO SALAD

Serves: **1**
Prep Time: **5** Minutes
Cook Time: **5** Minutes
Total Time: **10** Minutes

INGREDIENTS

- ¼ cooked quinoa
- ¼ cup avocado
- ¼ cup zucchini
- ¼ cup capsicum cubes
- ¼ cup mushroom
- ½ cup cherry tomatoes
- 1 cup lettuce
- 1 tablespoon sprouts
- 1 tsp olive oil
- Salad dressing

DIRECTIONS

1. **In a bowl combine all ingredients together**

2. Add salad dressing, toss well and serve

TOFU SALAD

Serves: *1*
Prep Time: *5* Minutes
Cook Time: *5* Minutes
Total Time: *10* Minutes

INGREDIENTS

- 1 pack tofu
- 1 cup chopped vegetables (carrots, cucumber)

DRESSING

- 1 tablespoon sesame oil
- 1 tablespoon mustard
- 1 tablespoon brown rice vinegar
- 1 tablespoon soya sauce

DIRECTIONS

1. In a bowl combine all ingredients together
2. Add salad dressing, toss well and serve

PAD THAI SALAD

Serves: 1
Prep Time: 5 Minutes
Cook Time: 5 Minutes
Total Time: 10 Minutes

INGREDIENTS

- ¼ lb. rice noodles
- 1 red pepper
- 1 onion
- 4 stalks coriander
- ¼ package silken tofu
- 1 oz. roasted peanuts
- Salad dressing

DIRECTIONS

1. In a bowl combine all ingredients together
2. Add salad dressing, toss well and serve

AVOCADO SALAD

Serves: **1**

Prep Time: **5** Minutes

Cook Time: **5** Minutes

Total Time: **10** Minutes

INGREDIENTS

- 2 avocados
- ¼ lb. snap peas
- 1 tablespoon sesame seeds

SALAD DRESSING

- 1 tablespoon soya sauce
- 1 tablespoon umeboshi puree
- 2 tablespoons mikawa mirin

DIRECTIONS

1. In a bowl combine all ingredients together
2. Add salad dressing, toss well and serve

MUSHROOM SALAD

Serves: *1*
Prep Time: *5* Minutes
Cook Time: *5* Minutes
Total Time: *10* Minutes

INGREDIENTS

- ½ lb. mushrooms
- 1 clove garlic
- ½ lb. salad leaves
- ¼ lb. tofu
- 1 oz. walnuts
- salad dressing

DIRECTIONS

1. In a bowl combine all ingredients together
2. Add salad dressing, toss well and serve

MIXED GREENS SALAD

Serves: **1**

Prep Time: **5** Minutes

Cook Time: **5** Minutes

Total Time: **10** Minutes

INGREDIENTS

- 2 cucumbers
- 3 radishes
- ¼ red bell pepper
- 2 spring onions
- 1 tablespoon red wine vinegar
- 1 tablespoon rice vinegar
- 1 tablespoon soya sauce
- 1 tablespoon clearspring mirin
- 2 cups mixed salad greens

DIRECTIONS

1. In a bowl combine all ingredients together
2. Add salad dressing, toss well and serve

QUINOA SALAD

Serves: **1**

Prep Time: **5** Minutes

Cook Time: **5** Minutes

Total Time: **10** Minutes

INGREDIENTS

- 1 cup cooked quinoa
- ¼ cup clearspring hijiki
- ¼ red bell pepper
- 1 bun watercress
- 2 radishes
- 2 tablespoons goji berries

DIRECTIONS

1. In a bowl combine all ingredients together
2. Add salad dressing, toss well and serve

DINNER

ONION SOUP

Serves: **4**

Prep Time: **10** Minutes

Cook Time: **20** Minutes

Total Time: **30** Minutes

INGREDIENTS

- 6 spring onions
- ½ red onion
- 1 potato
- 1 tablespoon olive oil
- Salt
- ¼ tsp coriander

DIRECTIONS

1. In a pot place the potatoes, water and boil until the potatoes are soft
2. In another pot heat olive oil and sauté spring onions and onion until soft

3. Add boiled potatoes to the pot where are the sauté onions
4. Add coriander, salt, pepper and stir well
5. Blend the soup until the soup is creamy
6. When ready pour into bowls and serve

ZUCCHINI SOUP

Serves: **6**
Prep Time: **10** Minutes
Cook Time: **25** Minutes
Total Time: **35** Minutes

INGREDIENTS

- 1 onion
- 1 tsp olive oil
- 1 zucchini
- 1 cup corn
- 1 cup broth
- 1 cup soy yogurt
- 1 tsp red pepper flakes
- 1 tablespoon cilantro
- 1 tablespoon parmesan

DIRECTIONS

1. In a skillet sauté onion until soft
2. Add zucchinis, corn and sauté for 5-6 minutes

3. Stir in water, vegetable broth, black pepper and salt
4. Bring everything to a boil and cook for 8-10 minutes
5. Add soy yogurt, cilantro, red pepper flakes and cook for another 5-6 minutes
6. When ready ad parmesan and serve

SAUERKRAUT SOUP

Serves: **4**

Prep Time: **10** Minutes

Cook Time: **30** Minutes

Total Time: **40** Minutes

INGREDIENTS

- 2 celery sticks
- 1 onion
- 2 carrots
- 2 potatoes
- 1 cup mushrooms
- 1 cup sauerkraut
- 6 cups vegetable broth
- 1 tablespoon olive oil
- 1 cup tofu
- 1 bay leaf

DIRECTIONS

1. **In a pot heat olive oil and add tofu**

2. Cook until crispy and set aside
3. Sauté onion and mushrooms for 2-3 minutes
4. Add vegetable broth and the rest of the ingredients
5. Bring everything to a boil and simmer on low heat for 18-20 minutes
6. When the soup is ready remove the bay leaf and transfer soup to a blender
7. Blend until smooth and serve with tofu slices on top

GREEK RICE SOUP

Serves: **6**

Prep Time: **10** Minutes

Cook Time: **35** Minutes

Total Time: **45** Minutes

INGREDIENTS

- 1 onion
- 1 carrot
- 1 cup celery
- 4 cups vegetable broth
- ¼ cup rice
- ½ cup tofu
- 1 tablespoon dill
- 1 lemon

EGG MIXTURE

- 1 cup coconut milk
- 1 cup tofu
- 2 tablespoons lemon juice
- 1 tsp salt

- 1 tsp black pepper
- 1 tsp nutritional yeast

DIRECTIONS

1. In a pot heat olive oil and add carrots, celery, onion and sauté until vegetables are soft
2. Add rice, vegetable broth and cook until the rice absorbs the liquid
3. In a blender add the ingredients for the egg mixture and blend until smooth
4. Pour the egg mixture into the soup and stir well
5. Add tofu, dill and any remaining ingredients to the soup
6. Cover and cook until the soup is ready

GAZPACHO

Serves: 2
Prep Time: 10 Minutes
Cook Time: 10 Minutes
Total Time: 20 Minutes

INGREDIENTS

- 1 cucumber
- ½ cup tomato juice
- 4 tomatoes
- ¼ avocado
- 1 garlic clove
- ¼ red onion
- 2 tablespoons red wine vinegar
- 1 tablespoon olive oil
- black pepper

DIRECTIONS

1. In a blender add all ingredients for the soup and blend until smooth

2. Pour soup in a container add seasoning and mix well
3. Serve when ready and refrigerate remaining soup

TORTELLINI SOUP

Serves: **6**

Prep Time: **10** Minutes

Cook Time: **20** Minutes

Total Time: **30** Minutes

INGREDIENTS

- 1 cup crushed tomatoes
- 3 cups vegetable broth
- 1 tsp tomato paste
- 1 tsp basil
- 1 tsp oregano
- 2 cups mushrooms tortellini
- 2 cups baby spinach

DIRECTIONS

1. In a pot sauté onion and garlic
2. Ad tofu and cook until soft
3. Add the rest of the ingredients to the pot and cook for another 10-12 minutes

4. Cook until tortellini are done
5. When ready remove soup from heat and serve

LEBANESE SOUP

Serves: **4**

Prep Time: **10** Minutes

Cook Time: **25** Minutes

Total Time: **35** Minutes

INGREDIENTS

- 1 tablespoon olive oil
- 1 onion
- 1 carrot
- 1 large potato
- 1 garlic clove
- 1 bay leaf
- 1 cup cooked chickpeas
- 1 tomato
- 2 cups vegetable broth
- 1 cup water
- 1 tablespoon tomato pate
- 1 tsp paprika
- 1 tablespoon parsley

DIRECTIONS

1. In a saucepan sauté garlic and onion
2. Add tomatoes, carrots, potatoes and cook for another 4-5 minutes
3. Add remaining ingredients and bring soup to a boil
4. Simmer on low heat for 15-18 minutes
5. When ready remove from heat and serve

BROCCOLI SOUP

Serves: **4**
Prep Time: **10** Minutes
Cook Time: **15** Minutes
Total Time: **25** Minutes

INGREDIENTS

- 2 lb. broccoli
- 2 potatoes
- 2 garlic cloves
- 1 onion
- 2 tablespoons nutritional yeast
- 1 tablespoon olive oil
- 1 tsp salt

DIRECTIONS

1. In a pot add potatoes, broccoli, onion and sauté until vegetables are soft
2. Place saluted veggies in a blender, add garlic, nutritional yeast, salt and blend until smooth
3. Add remaining ingredients and blend again

4. When ready transfer to a plate, drizzle olive oil and serve

SWEET POTATO SOUP

Serves: **4**

Prep Time: **10** Minutes

Cook Time: **30** Minutes

Total Time: **40** Minutes

INGREDIENTS

- 3 sweet potatoes
- 1 onion
- 2 carrots
- ¼ tsp cumin
- ¼ tsp red pepper
- olive oil
- 1-inch piece ginger
- water

DIRECTIONS

1. Place all vegetables in a pot
2. Add water and bring to a boil
3. Boil on low heat for 25-30 minutes

4. When vegetables are tender blend soup
5. Add remaining ingredients and blend again
6. Pour soup into a bowl, season and serve

VEGAN PHO

Serves: **6**

Prep Time: **10** Minutes

Cook Time: **35** Minutes

Total Time: **45** Minutes

INGREDIENTS

- 4 cups vegetable broth
- 1 package rice noodles
- 1 cup mushrooms
- 1 carrot
- 1 tablespoon coconut aminos
- 1 tsp sriracha
- 2 cloves garlic
- 1 onion
- 1 bunch cilantro
- 1 chili pepper
- 1-star anise
- handful of green onion

DIRECTIONS

1. In a saucepan heat coconut oil and add star-anise, vegetable broth, coconut aminos, sriracha and bring to a boil
2. Add soy sauce, vegetable broth and simmer on low heat for 20-25 minutes
3. In a frying pan fry mushrooms, add noodles, carrot, cilantro and fry for another 2-3 minutes
4. Add the fried vegetables to the soup and boil for 5-10 minutes
5. When ready remove from heat, pour into bowls and serve with green onions

SMOOTHIES

MACROBIOTIC SMOOTHIE

Serves: **1**
Prep Time: **5** Minutes
Cook Time: **5** Minutes
Total Time: **10** Minutes

INGREDIENTS

- 1 apple
- 2 bananas
- 2 packs acai
- ginger
- 1 cup ice

DIRECTIONS

1. In a blender place all ingredients and blend until **smooth**
2. Pour smoothie in a glass and serve

PALEO SMOOTHIE

Serves: **1**

Prep Time: **5** Minutes

Cook Time: **5** Minutes

Total Time: **10** Minutes

INGREDIENTS

- 2 bananas
- ½ cup blueberries
- 1 tsp spirulina powder
- 1 tablespoon almonds powder
- 1 cup almond milk
- 1 cup coconut milk
- 1 tablespoon coconut oil

DIRECTIONS

1. In a blender place all ingredients and blend until smooth
2. Pour smoothie in a glass and serve

MORNING CHOCHOLATE SMOOTHIE

Serves: *1*

Prep Time: *5* Minutes

Cook Time: *5* Minutes

Total Time: *10* Minutes

INGREDIENTS

- ½ cup spinach leaves
- 1 tablespoon mint
- 1 tablespoon cocoa powder
- 1 cup coconut milk
- 1 cup almond milk
- 1 cup ice

DIRECTIONS

1. **In a blender place all ingredients and blend until smooth**
2. **Pour smoothie in a glass and serve**

ALKALINE SMOOTHIE

Serves: **1**
Prep Time: **5** Minutes
Cook Time: **5** Minutes
Total Time: **10** Minutes

INGREDIENTS

- 1 cup almond milk
- 1 tablespoon ginger powder
- Juice of 1 grapefruit
- 1 avocado
- 1 tsp coconut oil
- ½ cucumber
- pinch of cinnamon
- 1 cub ice

DIRECTIONS

1. **In a blender place all ingredients and blend until smooth**
2. **Pour smoothie in a glass and serve**

SIMPLE MACROBIOTIC SMOOTHIE

Serves: *1*
Prep Time: 5 Minutes
Cook Time: 5 Minutes
Total Time: 10 Minutes

INGREDIENTS

- 1 tablespoon wakame seaweed
- 1 cup almond milk
- 1 green apple
- 1 carrot
- 1 cucumber
- 1 cup coconut milk
- 1 cup ice

DIRECTIONS

1. In a blender place all ingredients and blend until smooth
2. Pour smoothie in a glass and serve

ENERGY BOOSTING SMOOTHIE

Serves: **1**

Prep Time: **5** Minutes

Cook Time: **5** Minutes

Total Time: **10** Minutes

INGREDIENTS

- 1 cup coconut milk
- 1 grapefruit
- 1 lemon
- 1 tsp almond powder
- ¼ cup coconut flakes
- cinnamon
- ½ cup grapes

DIRECTIONS

1. In a blender place all ingredients and blend until smooth
2. Pour smoothie in a glass and serve

TURMERIC SMOOTHIE

Serves: *1*
Prep Time: *5* Minutes
Cook Time: *5* Minutes
Total Time: *10* Minutes

INGREDIENTS

- 1 handful of kale
- ½ cup pineapple
- 1 tsp turmeric
- ¼ tsp ginger
- 1 pinch pepper
- 1 spoon chia seeds
- 1 cup almond milk

DIRECTIONS

1. In a blender add all the ingredients and blend until smooth
2. Pour in a glass and serve

PINEAPPLE SMOOTHIE

Serves: **1**

Prep Time: **5** Minutes

Cook Time: **5** Minutes

Total Time: **10** Minutes

INGREDIENTS

- ½ pineapple
- 2 ribs celery
- 1 head romaine lettuce
- 1 handful coriander
- 1-inch ginger

DIRECTIONS

1. In a blender add all the ingredients and blend until smooth
2. Pour in a glass and serve

KIWI-KALE SMOOTHIE

Serves: **1**

Prep Time: **5** Minutes

Cook Time: **5** Minutes

Total Time: **10** Minutes

INGREDIENTS

- 4 oz. water
- 1 mango
- 1 kiwifruit
- 1 cup kale

DIRECTIONS

1. In a blender place all ingredients and blend until smooth
2. Pour smoothie in a glass and serve

STRAWBERRY SMOOTHIE

Serves: **1**
Prep Time: **5** Minutes
Cook Time: **5** Minutes
Total Time: **10** Minutes

INGREDIENTS

- 5 oz. water
- 1 banana
- 3 strawberries
- 1 orange
- 1 baby spinach

DIRECTIONS

1. **In a blender place all ingredients and blend until smooth**
2. **Pour smoothie in a glass and serve**

THANK YOU FOR READING THIS BOOK!

Made in the USA
Monee, IL
05 February 2024